Natural cosmetics DIY

Homemade beauty products

Fabienne Rausch

Introduction

In the midst of the discussion about environmental protection, recycling and sustainability, an ever-growing group has developed in the background that has come up with the idea of also making cosmetic products themselves, vegan and with as little waste as possible. In the meantime, there are a large number of recipes for the most diverse products. From simple hand cream to make-up and nail polish to homemade hair treatments, you can actually make everything yourself. Homemade cosmetics are not only better for the environment, but your skin and hair also benefit from fewer chemical products and are cared for with purely natural or sometimes even animal products.

In this book, you will find different recipes for a variety of everyday cosmetic products that you can make yourself, and there are also tips or explanations about individual ingredients or sustainable options. For most recipes you only need a few ingredients and since a few ingredients are suitable as the basis of most recipes, you can build up a small stock. Coconut oil, essential oils, shea butter or vegetable oils like olive oil actually appear in almost every recipe. So if you like to switch to a homemade alternative for several cosmetic products, you can buy a larger pack right away.

In addition to the recipe suggestions listed here, you can also find a wide range of different ideas on the internet and with a little experience you can also develop your own recipes. If you need certain ingredients or want to make a cream with a certain active ingredient, you can also ask for advice in a drugstore or search the internet for plants that contain this active ingredient. In this way, you can not only make nourishing cosmetic products yourself, but also, among other things, ointments with a pain-relieving or anti-inflammatory effect, face masks with an anti-aging effect or hair treatments with a strengthening effect. It is not always necessary to use chemical products to achieve good effects; purely natural products usually have a much better effect and are also much gentler to use.

By the way, homemade soaps, creams or perfumes are also a great gift idea and not only for Christmas, but also for birthdays, special occasions or just as a great present. Together with a beautiful packaging, a special colour combination or an individual scent, you can make every gift an eye-catcher and surely everyone is happy about such a sustainable and homemade gift.

DIY cosmetics

1. Soap

There are many different variations for making your own soap. Besides the difference between solid and liquid soap, you can also choose whether you want to make the raw soap yourself or whether you prefer to buy it. The finished soap is not only excellent as a small gift for birthdays or Christmas, but also unbeatable in terms of sustainability. The homemade soap contains only the ingredients you want to put in it, you can get creative with the smell and look and really let off steam for once.

Making your own soap is not that difficult and most of the ingredients you need are probably already in your bathroom or kitchen cupboard. The additional ingredients usually don't cost much and are available in every drugstore, so you can always decide spontaneously to start making your own soap.

As already mentioned, there are two main differences in making and you need to consider at the beginning whether you want to start a "last minute" action or if you have a bit of time and also make the raw soap yourself. If you are in a hurry, you can easily buy raw soap on Amazon or in the drugstore and there you can even choose between different types made from goat's milk, with shea butter or as transparent soap. The other option takes a few weeks longer, but you can really talk about 100% homemade soap afterwards.

Homemade soap with bought raw soap

Ingredients:
- ♥ Raw soap
- ♥ Soap colour
- ♥ Fragrance oil
- ♥ Ingredients for decorating, for example flower petals, dried lemon, coffee...

To make this soap, you first need to melt the raw soap slowly in a water bath over a medium heat, stirring all the time so that nothing settles to the bottom of the bowl. Once the soap is completely liquid, you can go wild and add colour and fragrance oil as desired. Depending on the desired look, you can also divide the liquid soap into several small bowls and use different shades to colour it. Before you fill the soap into your desired form, you can add other ingredients to give it a very personal look. Depending on the scent, a few lavender flowers, dried lemon slices or flower petals are suitable for example.

The mould does not necessarily have to be a soap mould, simple silicone moulds or baking tins are also particularly suitable. You can take a look in your kitchen cupboard and see which mould you like best. The only important thing is that you get the soap out of the mould safely, so that all the decoration is not wasted in the end because you can no longer get the soap out.

If you have chosen different shades, you can also pull a toothpick or fork through the soap and mix the different colours slightly to create a beautiful colour gradient. This creates a beautiful marble pattern and you don't just have two blobs of colour next to each other.

After the soap has set well, you can then turn the mould over and cut the soap into final pieces, wrap it up nicely or put it straight into the bath and try it out straight away. If you want to make more soap at once and don't have enough small moulds, you can simply pour the mixture into a larger cake mould and then cut it into smaller pieces. However, the soap may take a few hours longer to cool down, so it is better to wait two to three hours longer.

Homemade soap with your own raw soap	Ingredients: ♥ 650g coconut fat (hardened) ♥ 650g sunflower oil ♥ 650g olive oil (clear, not naturally cloudy) ♥ 290g caustic soda (sodium hydroxide) ♥ 1 litre mineral water

For this recipe, you need to allow a little more time, because before making the actual soap, you first need to let the raw soap mature for about 30 days. However, to avoid having to start all over again and wait a month, you can also make a larger quantity of the raw soap and store it in a dry and cool place. The ingredients listed here are enough for about 2kg of raw soap and of course you can start with a smaller amount first to try everything out.

The first step is to put the coconut oil and the oil together in a pot and heat it slowly to about 35 degrees. It is best to check the temperature with a stick thermometer every now and then so that the mixture does not get too hot.

At the same time, you can weigh out the caustic soda in a plastic bag, which you must dispose of afterwards, as caustic soda is not suitable for eating and should not come into contact with food. This lye is then tipped into a sufficiently large bucket with the water, making sure that you pour in the water first and then add the lye. When the lye is added, the water heats up considerably and may even boil over and produce hot vapours. It is best to do this step either in the open air or at an open window so that nothing can happen. You should also stand as far away as possible when pouring the water together and ideally wear gloves and goggles so that you can protect yourself and do not scald yourself with boiling water or similar.

Once both mixtures are ready, you have to check the temperature regularly and wait for the moment when both solutions have reached about 35°C. If the temperature is not right when you pour them together, the saponification will not work, and all the work will be in vain. If the temperature is not right when pouring together, the desired saponification will not work, and all the work will have been in vain. So, it is better to wait a few minutes longer before you have to start all over again.

If the temperature is right, you can pour the two liquids together while stirring constantly and continue stirring until the mixture becomes more solid and the spoon draws traces. However, as this can take a long time, you can take an old food processor to help you and slowly run a stirrer through the soap on the lowest setting.

Finally, you can put the soap on a baking tray or in a mould to let it harden for a few days. When pouring the soap and stirring it, be careful that the lye is still corrosive at that moment and should never come into contact with bare skin. Again, gloves and long clothes are required and if you are starting soap production together with children, it is good if they take over this step. You should then wrap the mould with a few towels so that the heat is released as evenly as possible and thus the shape and structure are retained.

After three to four days, when the soap has set well, you can cut it into small cubes with a knife or a spatula and leave it to harden for another three weeks. During this time, you can always check how far along the raw soap is with a pH test, because the optimal pH value should be between 5.5 and 10. Very skin-friendly soaps usually have a value of 7.5 to 8.5 and you can of course also make different soaps with different pH values.

From raw soap to soap

Once the first step is done, it is now a matter of refining the soap with the desired fragrance and decorating it a little or giving it a different shape. Compared to the first step, refining is very easy and much quicker. All you have to do is cut the raw soap into small pieces, heat them over a water bath and add the desired ingredients. Then you put the liquid into the desired shape, let it cool and your soap is ready to use.

Fruity lemon soap for the summer

For this variation, in addition to 500g of raw soap, you need two to three lemons, 25g of lemon oil and a little yellow soap colour. Cut the lemons into narrow strips a few days before you actually make the soap and leave them to dry in a dry and airy place until all the moisture has evaporated. Of course, you can also skip this step by buying already dried lemon slices and using them for decorating. Then melt the raw soap in a water bath and add the lemon oil. If you're wondering at this point why simple lemon juice won't work, here's the answer right away. Although the juice certainly smells just as intense and seems to be a good and, above all, sustainable alternative at first glance, the smell dissipates much more quickly and after just a few times, neither the soap nor your hands will really smell of lemon.

Once you have mixed everything, add the yellow colour at the end. You should proceed gradually and add a few drops at a time until you have reached the desired colour. Otherwise, you run the risk of the soap looking unnatural and a very bright yellow.

While the mixture is still on the cooker, you can grease your mould and position the lemon slices as desired. You can also add more slices as an intermediate layer when filling the soap or press in a final lemon slice on top. Then place the finished mould in a cool place where the soap can harden for two to three days, depending on its thickness, before you turn it out and add the finishing touches.

Besides lemon, you can of course choose many other scents and follow the same steps. Maybe you prefer the smell of lavender, cinnamon or coconut, or you want to try out some crazy recipes and mix coffee or espresso powder into the soap, for example. Depending on the intensity you want, you can also use a little less or more fragrance oil and especially with spice fragrances, the spices themselves are also very suitable.

-Vegan and Sustainable-

For particularly sustainable soap, you should definitely look for fair trade when buying the products and, if possible, also buy regionally. In addition, many colours can be made yourself and you can also use beetroot, coffee powder, turmeric or similar instead of the industrially produced soap colours. Of course, you should make sure that the smell of the soap does not change significantly, but otherwise there is nothing to be said against using homemade colouring agents. Stir in the appropriate powder like the soap colour and mix everything well so that there are no lumps or large dark colour spots.

Soap is actually vegan in most cases, especially with homemade raw soap you are on the safe side. However, if you want to buy the raw soap, you should of course pay attention to the ingredients and avoid products with goat's milk, beeswax or honey. Honey or milk powder is also out of the question when it comes to refining, but there are enough natural products to create a pleasant smell and a nice washing sensation.

2. Face cream

Ingredients:
- ♥ 1/2 cup shea butter
- ♥ 2 tsp nourishing oil (coconut oil, jojoba oil, avocado oil, almond oil, etc.)
- ♥ 10 drops essential oil
- ♥ Water

It is often not easy to find the right face cream for your skin type and in many cases the skin reacts irritably to the many chemical additives and the desired effect is not achieved. But fortunately, making face creams is not that difficult and with just a few ingredients you can create your very own individual cream for your skin type. You can decide for yourself which ingredients to choose and which you would rather leave out. You may even know from experience that your skin is sensitive to certain substances and can avoid them. Making the face cream is really super easy and you only need four ingredients for the basic recipe.

First, heat the shea butter and oil together in a water bath to about 60 degrees, being careful not to raise the temperature too high too quickly. You can also boil the water at the same time; the amount can vary slightly depending on the desired consistency. Before you can add the two liquids together, the water must be cooled down again to 60 degrees so that the ingredients have the same temperature. While stirring, you can then gradually add a little water until you get a nice creamy consistency that is not too runny. While stirring, the cream also cools down at the same time, which allows you to judge the consistency even better. Once the cream has been stirred and cooled, you can add the essential oil to give the face cream a pleasant fragrance. You can then pour the finished product into a suitable and clean jar with a lid and ideally consume it within the next three to four months.

This face cream is suitable for all skin types and it not only moisturises, but also makes the skin look fresher and younger. Whether you put it on your face before you go to sleep or do it after, the effect is always very intense, and you will be surprised how much better and fitter you feel afterwards.

3. Make-up

Make-up often not only costs a lot of money but is also not so good for the environment and in many products, you can read a number of chemical products in the ingredients list. But in the future, you can do without the chemical additives, animal testing and waste of resources by simply making your own mascara, song shadow or make-up remover. One advantage of this is that you can always make the right amount and if you know you don't need that much, you can just make half of it before the rest ends up dried out in the trash.

<u>Mascara</u>

Ingredients:
- ♥ Xanthan gum
- ♥ 1 teaspoon of healing clay
- ♥ 1 teaspoon activated charcoal
- ♥ 1 teaspoon grain or vodka
- ♥ 1/2 teaspoon aloe vera gel

Mascara is probably the make-up product that is used most often, but unfortunately also dries up most often. To ensure that you always have the right amount of mascara on hand in the future and can even save dried-up mascara, here is a simple recipe that can be tried out quickly.

First, put all the dry ingredients together in a bowl and mix everything together well before adding some aloe vera gel and vodka / grain. It is best to stir in the liquid as quickly as possible so that no large lumps form and the mascara doesn't end up looking more like a peel. If you feel that you need a little more liquid, you can also gradually add more vodka and aloe vera gel.

You can either put the finished mascara in an old and washed-out mascara bottle, or in a small, sealable jar and place a matching brush separately. You can also use old and washed-out containers for the brushes; you don't necessarily have to buy new ones. By the way, if the mascara dries out, you can simply add a few drops of vodka, mix everything together and you have liquid and functioning mascara again.

Powder without plastic

Powder is easy to make with just a few household products. In addition, you also have the option of choosing a more intense or matte colour depending on your skin type. To make the powder, all you need is some corn starch, healing clay and varying amounts of cocoa or cinnamon, depending on the desired colour. The smell of the two powders dissipates on the skin, so you don't have to worry about smelling like cinnamon afterwards. Simply mix all the ingredients together until you get a powder with a uniform colour and apply some to your skin to test. If it is still too light, you can stir in more cocoa powder or cinnamon, but if it is too dark, you can add more corn starch.

Ingredients:
- ♥ 2 teaspoons cornflour
- ♥ 1 to 2 teaspoons of healing clay (e.g. Luvos haut fein, available in every drugstore).
- ♥ 0.5 to 1 teaspoon cinnamon powder or cocoa powder for baking

The cinnamon powder has other advantages besides its colouring function, because it has an invigorating and antibacterial effect on the skin. Not only does it make you look fresher, but the cinnamon powder also fights against impurities and bacteria, so you also have a kind of mask included in the powder.

Quick make-up remover

To remove the make-up at the end of the day, natural make-up remover is the best and most effective option. There is a wide range of simple ways to make the right product yourself. For example, you can use commercially available coconut oil by first moistening your face a little and then going over it with a small portion of coconut oil. Massage the oil in a little, but make sure to be a little more careful around the eyes or just use a cotton pad. Once you have distributed everything nicely, you can wash the oil off again directly and you will not only have removed your make-up, but you will also have cared for your skin and given it a new freshness. In addition to coconut oil, aloe vera gel is also suitable, which has a similar nourishing effect and thus makes an additional face cream unnecessary.

4. Body lotion

As with face cream, it is often complicated to find the right product for body lotion, and in the end, you don't use it at all because there is simply nothing that is right for you. But fortunately, there are now a few ways to make your own body lotion. This way, you can do without animal testing and chemicals. However, there are several different ways to make body lotion. You can choose between an emulsion, which is a mixture of fat and water, or a body butter, which is made without water. Both types are very effective, but in the end, you have to decide for yourself which is better for you and your skin.

Body butter

Ingredients:
- ♥ 20 g virgin coconut oil
- ♥ 10 g shea butter
- ♥ 15 g cocoa butter
- ♥ 5 g olive oil

The basic ingredients for the body butter are almost identical to the ingredients for the face cream and here too, coconut oil and shea butter are first heated slowly over a water bath. However, 15g of cocoa butter is added, which is also heated over a water bath before the olive oil is slowly stirred into the mixture.

When the cream is ready, you can add different essential oils to get the desired scent. For example, the variant with vanilla aroma smells very good, but rose oil, lemon scent or honey are also suitable. Again, try and try until you find your perfect fragrance. The mixture is then placed in the refrigerator to cool for about 30 minutes, after which you can use a blender or mixer to loosen up the cream again and bring it to the right consistency. Finally, pour the body butter into a small jar. You can store it in a dark and cool place for a few months. Alternatively, you can freeze the cream in portions in ice cube moulds and defrost as needed. This preserves the moisture better and you can also make a larger quantity at a time without fear of the cream going bad too quickly.

Body Lotion with Aloe Vera

Ingredients:
- ♥ 50 ml cold-pressed organic coconut oil
- ♥ 50 ml aloe vera gel

For this recipe, you really only need two ingredients and little time to make a good body lotion. All you need to do is put both ingredients together in a blender, mix well and then store in a jar in a cool, dark place.

You can even make the required aloe vera gel yourself by peeling a leaf of aloe vera and then finely pureeing it. Since the plant itself already brings fragrance, you don't even need a fragrance oil or aroma to make the lotion smell good. If the body lotion is too liquid for you, you can change the ratio of oil and gel a little by adding more coconut oil or using a little less aloe vera gel. Before you do this, make sure that you have mixed the cream well, because the water content in the aloe vera gel can make it a little more difficult to mix the two ingredients at the beginning. To be on the safe side, you can also let the body lotion rest for a while and then see if the consistency is right or if you need to change something.

Cleopatra Body Lotion

Ingredients:
- ♥ 50 ml milk
- ♥ 100 ml almond oil
- ♥ 0.5 tsp honey
- ♥ 10 drops of essential oil of choice

Even in Egypt, people knew that the mixture of milk and honey had a positive effect on the skin and so this body lotion also provides a lot of moisture and works against wrinkles. Due to the milk, in which the emulsion of fat and water has already taken place, all ingredients mix without any problems. This means that there is no danger of the oil or honey settling over time.

To mix the ingredients, first whip the milk with a hand blender in a high appliance. Then you can slowly add the almond oil and stir it in carefully but quickly with the mixer. Finally, add half a teaspoon of honey and if you would like a little more fragrance, you can add a few drops of an essential oil. Once everything is well mixed, you can pour the body lotion back into a small container and use it up within the next few months or give it as a gift. Although the oil and honey make the milk last a little longer, it is best to store the body lotion in the fridge and not keep it for too long. The freezing method is again possible here and if you have made a larger quantity, you can simply put some in ice cube moulds and place in the freezer.

Body lotion against cellulite

Ingredients:
- ♥ 35 g shea butter
- ♥ 35 g coconut oil
- ♥ 25 g almond oil
- ♥ 5 drops cedar oil
- ♥ 5 drops rosemary oil
- ♥ 5 drops orange oil

Many people struggle with annoying cellulite and try many things to finally get rid of it. Perhaps you are one of them and are grateful for every tip that helps you to make cellulite disappear. Of course, this body lotion will not work miracles overnight and make all your cellulite go away. However, the essential oils help in the fight against cellulite and gradually reduce it.

To make the body lotion, first heat the shea butter and coconut oil slowly in a water bath and then carefully stir in the almond oil. Once everything is nicely combined, you can add the essential oils and mix everything well one more time. Then put everything in the fridge for half an hour so that the mixture can set well. After that, you can mix the body lotion with a blender until it has the desired consistency and is pleasant for you. Bottled in a clean and sealable jar, the cream will keep for about four weeks. Again, you can use the freezer trick to keep the cream for longer. Below you will find a small list of typical ingredients for body lotions and their helpful effects. Most ingredients have several positive effects, of course, but mainly the ones mentioned here. These are also the reasons for using them in body, hand or face creams.

Almond oil, sandalwood oil	✓ moisturising
Rose water	✓ antibacterial effect
Cedar oil	✓ Stimulates the lymphatic flow & ensures drainage→ thus helps against cellulite & tightens the skin
Rosemary oil	✓ Drains & stimulates blood circulation
Orange essential oil	✓ Tightens weak connective tissue
Coconut oil	✓ Provides moisture ✓ Has an antibacterial effect & prevents blemished skin
Lavender oil	✓ Promotes blood circulation ✓ Soothes the skin
Olive oil	✓ Provides moisture
Aloe Vera Gel	✓ Ensures quick absorption of the body lotion ✓ anti-inflammatory, antibacterial, antiviral, firming effect
Beeswax	✓ Forms a protective film on the skin that prevents skin irritation ✓ Provides moisture
Shea butter	✓ Provides dry skin with moisture ✓ has a calming & moisturising effect
Cocoa butter	✓ Melts well on the skin, therefore easily spreadable ✓ Leaves skin silky ✓ moisturising
Vanilla oil	✓ Promotes blood circulation ✓ anti-inflammatory effect

5. Foot cream

Feet have to endure a lot every day and especially in winter they are far too dry. And then there is the callus on the heels that tears. Everyone knows the problem of dry feet and in search of a good antidote you have certainly tried one or the other cream. Homemade foot creams are also very good, especially if you want to reach for vegan and sustainable products without animal testing, you should definitely give them a try.

There are many different types of foot creams, not only to buy, but also to make yourself, and while some of them help especially with dry feet, there are also warming creams or those against calluses. So it is best to think about what the cream is for and what effect you want to achieve before you make it.

Foot cream for dry and cracked feet

Ingredients:
- 20 g lanolin anhydride
- 20 ml shea butter
- 2.5 g urea powder
- 4 g beeswax
- essential oils

A good foot cream is especially urgently needed when your feet are already a bit cracked, and you want to prevent the cracks from becoming inflamed or the dry skin from tearing even further. To do your feet some good in such situations, you can use this cream, which is particularly effective thanks to the lanolin anhydride. Lanolin is contained in many creams and ointments but can also be bought as such and thus mixed in even with creams. If you don't find what you are looking for in your local drugstore, ask at your local pharmacy, they will certainly be able to help you.

To make the cream, first put the lanolin anhydride, shea butter and beeswax in a water bath and let it melt slowly. At the same time, mix the urea powder with 40 ml of hot water and stir carefully until the powder is completely dissolved. When both are ready, you can take the bowl out of the water bath and gradually stir in the urea solution. To ensure that the cream has the right consistency, continue stirring until the mixture is about lukewarm and you can easily reach in. Finally, you can also add a few drops of an essential oil so that the foot cream smells more intense. Once everything is ready, put the cream back into a sealable jar and keep it in the fridge or another cool place and use it within the next month.

Foot butter for very dry feet

Ingredients:
- ♥ 8 grams grated beeswax
- ♥ 200 gram rose oil
- ♥ Possibly 10 drops of essential rose oil

For particularly dry feet, this rich foot butter is a "must have". Especially if you cream your feet before going to sleep and let the butter absorb overnight, it unfolds its full effect.

Due to the few ingredients, the foot butter is also very easy to make, because after you have melted the beeswax in a water bath, you can stir in the remaining ingredients directly. If you would prefer a different scent instead of the rose scent, you can also use alternative oils such as olive oil or coconut oil. In this case, however, you add the coconut oil to the water bath while it is melting and then just mix the desired essential oil with everything. Filled in a boiled and sealable jar, this foot butter will even keep for a whole year, although you should make sure it is stored in a cool place.

Warmth with ginger and apple

Ingredients:
- ♥ 100 ml boiled tap water
- ♥ 100 ml vegetable oil, e.g. coconut oil, olive oil or sesame oil
- ♥ 10 g beeswax
- ♥ 10 g Tegomuls (as emulsifier)
- ♥ a small apple
- ♥ 15 g ginger
- ♥ 2-3 pinches of cinnamon powder

The warming effect of this cream is achieved by active ingredients in apple, ginger and cinnamon, which first have to be dissolved in the oil. To do this, peel the apple and ginger, core the apple and then cut both into small pieces or use a grater to get really fine pieces. Then put the oil together with the cinnamon powder, ginger and apple in a small saucepan and let it simmer gently on a low heat. It should by no means boil too much, but, just barely, small bubbles should rise.

After 30 minutes, you can let everything cool down a bit and then pour it through a sieve so that the oil separates from the ginger and apple pieces. To get as much of the oil as possible, let it drain for a long time. Optionally, you can also squeeze out the remains in the sieve with a small spoon.

Now you just have to make the actual cream, and this actually works like any other cream. First, heat the oily ingredients together with the tegomuls, which you can find in a well-stocked drugstore or online, in a water bath to about 60 degrees. On the side, you can also boil the water and let it stand until it has reached a temperature of about 60 degrees again. Now, while still stirring, add the water to the fatty ingredients and keep stirring until you get a creamy consistency. If you don't feel like stirring the cream for a long time, you can also use a hand blender, which is much faster.

Finally, it is time to bottle it again and store it in a cool place. It is best to use the cream within the first two weeks. So, if you are planning the warming ointment as a gift, it is best to make it as soon as possible so that it can still be used for as long as possible.

6. Face masks/peelings

Especially the skin on the face is always causing problems and due to the daily stress caused by sweat, make-up and the like, good care is especially important. A good combination of good effect and little effort are definitely face masks and they come in all kinds. Whether against pimples, for firmer skin or as a moisturiser, a quickly made face mask always helps and is always ready.

Avocado against dry skin

Ingredients:
♥   ½ ripe avocado
♥   1-2 tbsp natural yoghurt
♥   1 tsp honey

This moisturising face mask is particularly easy to make, and you may even have all the ingredients for it at home.
All you have to do is mash half the avocado with a fork and then stir in the yoghurt and honey. Of course, you can also use vegan alternatives, because the mask also works perfectly with soy yoghurt and vegan honey.
Due to the high fat content of the avocado, its flesh is particularly suitable for dry and stressed skin. To use, simply apply the mask generously to your face and let it absorb for about ten to 15 minutes. Now just rinse the mask off with lukewarm water and lightly pat your face dry with a towel. After just one application, you can feel the soothing effect of the avocado on your skin, and you will notice that your skin is significantly better supplied with blood and also looks beautifully soft and fresh.

As this mask is not suitable for keeping for a longer period of time, it is best to make only the required amount at a time. However, due to the few ingredients and the simple preparation, this is not a problem and you can always make a small amount again if needed.

With protein against large pores

Ingredients:
- ♥ 1 egg white
- ♥ 1 teaspoon orange juice (freshly squeezed)
- ♥ 1/2 teaspoon turmeric powder

Large pores are just annoying, and you would prefer to get rid of them as soon as possible. Thanks to this face mask with egg white and orange juice, this is also easily possible, and you will already feel a visible change after two to three applications.

Mix one egg white with a dash of freshly squeezed orange juice and half a teaspoon of turmeric powder until you get an evenly coloured mask. The egg white works particularly well on oily pores, helping to shrink them and reduce excess oil production. The additional shot of vitamin C from the orange juice supports the effect and also ensures fresher and softer skin.

However, since turmeric is very colour-intensive, you should wear an old T-shirt when mixing the mask, as well as when applying it and letting it soak in, and it is not a problem if it gets the odd stain. After the exposure time, you can carefully rinse the mask off again with lukewarm water and gently pat your face dry. You can also store this mask in the fridge for a few days as long as it is hermetically sealed. Before use, stir everything vigorously once more so that the ingredients combine well.

Banana mask

Ingredients:
- 1 ripe banana
- 1 tsp honey

Just as simple and with a similar effect as the avocado mask, this banana mask is a real miracle cure for dry and stressed skin. Bananas also have a high fat content and together with the honey they provide a lot of moisture and make the skin look fresher again. You can either mash the banana finely with a fork or mash it briefly to create an even and slightly creamy mass. Before applying, add the honey, whereby a liquid honey is particularly suitable here. Now you only have to leave the mask on for about ten minutes and you can rinse it off with lukewarm water and admire the result.

Soothing honey mask for reddened skin

Ingredients:
- 2 tablespoons pure honey
- 1 teaspoon cinnamon
- 1 piece of fresh lemon

Reddened skin is not only a sign of dryness, but is often the

Inflammation is also associated with it and with this mask you can successfully combat the inflammation and redness. Cinnamon is known to reduce such inflammation and also fight against excess oil films.

For the mask, you can heat the honey briefly in a water bath or in the microwave so that it is nice and liquid and you can then stir in cinnamon and a dash of lemon juice without any problems. When everything has mixed well, you can apply the mask directly to the skin and massage it in for a few minutes like an exfoliator. After you have left the mask to work for about 15 minutes, you can rinse it off again with lukewarm water and lightly pat it dry.

You can also keep this mask refrigerated for a day or two, but then you should put it in the microwave or in a water bath for a short time so that it is nice and creamy again and everything mixes well. It would be best to make the mask fresh when needed, but as a small gift or if you are short of time, it can also be kept in the fridge for a while.

Ingredients:
- ♥ 2 tbsp. healing clay
- ♥ warm water

Fight against pimples and impurities with healing clay

Pimples and blemishes are always a nuisance. You just want to get rid of them as quickly as possible. As a natural aid without any chemicals, healing clay is perfect for this. This clay not only reduces inflammation, it also helps against itching and redness and at the same time binds excess sebum and bacteria. It is therefore a real all-rounder among face masks and is also very easy to make.

The healing clay, which is available in every drugstore and also in well-stocked supermarkets, only needs to be mixed with a little lukewarm water until a creamy and thick mass is formed. With this, you can start applying the mask to your face, avoiding the eye and mouth area. When the mask is completely dry, you can carefully wash it off with lukewarm water and you are done. As you should let the mask dry out completely, you should be really careful when adding water and make sure that the mask does not become too liquid. If necessary, you can always add some healing clay until the right consistency is reached again.

With this mask, it is no problem to store it for a longer period of time and you should only choose a cool and dark place for it. If you have made several portions, you can simply put the rest in a small jar, close it well and put it in a suitable place. The next time you use it, you may have to add a little more water, but otherwise nothing is missing, and the effect is definitely maintained.

The "recycling mask" made from coffee grounds

Ingredients:
- ♥ 5 tsp coffee grounds
- ♥ 1 tsp honey
- ♥ 1 tsp olive oil

Not only as a drink is coffee a real pick-me-up, but also in face masks, coffee grounds promote blood circulation and refresh the skin. So, the next time you make yourself a coffee, make sure you save some of the coffee grounds and mix it with some honey and olive oil. This combination is not only a face mask, but also an exfoliator, so it not only promotes circulation, but also provides a natural skin colour and removes small flakes, oil and sebum.

For application, you can slowly massage the mask into the skin with light circular movements. Again, it is best to avoid the eye and mouth area and apply more to the other areas. Once the mask has been evenly massaged in, you can leave it to work for about half an hour and rinse it off with lukewarm water.

Beyond these six masks, there are of course many more face masks that are super easy to make yourself and will significantly improve your skin's appearance. There are many more recipes on the internet, and at the same time you can also be inspired by products from the drugstore. However, you should not make face masks too often and especially if you have very irritated skin, it is better to do without them once in a while and give your skin a little rest first.

7. Body scrub

Peelings help the skin to circulate properly again and to free it from dandruff and the like. Simply massage it gently into the skin after showering, rinse it off with lukewarm water after a short time and the soothing peeling is ready. Of course, you can also use the peeling independently of showering, but here are a few tips. To make the peeling work especially well, you can prepare your skin before applying it and, for example, hold your face over a hot water bath. The steam opens the pores and activates the blood circulation, so that the subsequent peeling can remove sebum, bacteria and dandruff particularly efficiently. The basic ingredient of these scrubs is usually white or brown sugar, but you can also make one or two scrubs with sea salt.

Basic Sugar Scrub with Lemon

This peeling recipe is considered the basis and, depending on your mood, you can also refine it with other scents and essential oils. Basically, the peeling can be used on legs, arms and also on the face, although you have to be careful there that nothing gets into the eyes or nose.

Ingredients:
- ♥ 150 g sugar
- ♥ 50 g coconut oil
- ♥ 1/2 organic lemon
- ♥ 2 tbsp olive oil

To make it, first put the coconut oil in a water bath or in the microwave until it is completely liquid. At the same time, you can grate the zest from the lemon and then squeeze out the juice. Both things are then mixed with the sugar and the liquid oil until you get an even consistency. However, it should not be too liquid; if necessary, you can add a little more sugar.

Depending on how much and where you use the peeling, the amount is enough for about four servings and can be stored for several weeks without any problems. To do this, put the finished peeling in a sealable jar and store it in a cool place. Due to the high sugar content, it cannot actually go bad, but the lemon will eventually lose its refreshing effect.

Sea salt scrub

This recipe is again a basic recipe and can be modified as needed with different essential oils, lemon zest, cinnamon powder, coffee grounds or similar.

Ingredients:
- ♥ 500 g Dead Sea salt
- ♥ 250 ml almond oil
- ♥ essential oil

There is actually hardly any difference to the sugar scrub in the production, only the oil is already liquid from the start, which means you do not have to heat it up first. This means that sea salt and oil can be mixed directly and blended into an even scrub. The ratio is 2 to 1 and you should use about twice as much salt as oil. It is best not to tip everything together completely straight away but leave some oil so that you can weigh it out depending on the consistency. If the scrub is too dry, you can add more oil and vice versa, just add some more salt.

This scrub is also ready and waiting to be filled into small jars. Since salt is also an almost non-perishable foodstuff, you can store the scrub without any problems. For best results, however, you should use it within the first two months. The amount indicated is considerably more and is intended primarily for peeling lovers. If you want to be cautious and try out different recipes, you can also use only half or a fifth of the indicated amount.

The special winter peeling for Christmas

Ingredients:

- ♥ 100 g white sugar
- ♥ 100 g brown sugar
- ♥ 60 g coconut oil
- ♥ 2 tsp almond oil
- ♥ 1 tsp cocoa powder
- ♥ 1 tsp gingerbread spice
- ♥ 5 drops vanilla essential oil

Especially in winter, the skin is constantly stressed by the dry and cold air. A good smelling cinnamon peeling is the perfect way to do something really good for your skin. It also makes an excellent Christmas gift, and everyone is sure to be happy about such a peeling.

Although the recipe seems a little more complicated at first glance due to the longer ingredient list, you certainly already have most of the ingredients at home and the production actually works according to the same pattern. The division into brown and white sugar is also optional and only intended for layering in small gift jars.

As always, start by slowly heating the coconut oil on the cooker or in the microwave until it is completely liquid. In parallel, you can mix the white and brown sugar each with half of the other ingredients. You can also swap the essential oil for vanilla sugar or some vanilla paste if you don't want to buy an oil especially for this scrub. When the coconut oil is ready, you can divide the amount evenly between the two bowls and stir it in well. This scrub is rather dry, but you can add more coconut oil if you prefer it a little moister. Once you've mixed everything together nicely, you can now layer the brown and white sugar alternately in jars to create a nice striped pattern. The perfect Christmas gift is ready and of course it will look much nicer in your own bathroom cabinet.

8. Hand cream

Making a classic hand cream, as you can buy them, is usually comparatively complex and it takes a lot of patience and skill to get the emulsion right. Fortunately, there are much simpler recipes that use far fewer ingredients and achieve at least as good an effect.

Basic recipe

Ingredients:
- ♥ 160 g coconut oil
- ♥ 140 g shea butter / cocoa butter

The simplest recipe with only two ingredients is the mixture of coconut oil and shea butter. All you have to do is heat the shea butter in a water bath and then mix it with the coconut oil until it has a creamy and even consistency. The hand cream is ready and can be refined with different essential oils, depending on your choice. If you feel that the consistency is still too solid or too liquid even after cooling, you can either add a little shea butter or coconut oil until the hand cream has the right consistency.

Aloe Vera Cream

Ingredients:
- ♥ 100g Aloe Vera Gel
- ♥ 100g coconut oil / olive oil

For this recipe, which is also very simple, you need 100g of aloe vera gel in addition to the coconut oil, which you can also make yourself from an aloe vera leaf. All you have to do is "peel" the leaf so that you only have the almost transparent and gel-like inner part. Then put it into the blender until you have an even gel and there are no more pieces. When the gel is ready, you can add the melted coconut oil or olive oil to the blender and blend on high speed until you get a smooth cream. This creates an emulsion and the water from the aloe vera gel combines with the oil to form an even cream. When storing the hand cream, it can happen that the oil separates from the gel again over time and two different layers form, but these can quickly be blended again with the mixer to form a uniform emulsion.

The super cream for particularly dry skin

Ingredients:
- ♥ 50 ml almond oil
- ♥ 30 g coconut oil
- ♥ 20 g cocoa butter
- ♥ 5g beeswax
- ♥ optionally a few drops of tea tree oil (has an antibacterial effect)

Especially in winter, you often need a lot of good hand cream to protect your hands from drying out and to keep them moisturised despite the cold and dry air. If you add some beeswax to the hand cream, it has a much more intensive effect and provides more moisture than classic creams.

Again, the preparation is very simple and after you have liquefied all the solid ingredients in a water bath, you can stir in the almond oil and optionally add some tea tree oil. This gives your hand cream a second effect, because tea tree oil has an antibacterial effect and thus protects against inflammation in chapped areas on the one hand, but also against colds on the other. Once you have mixed everything into a smooth cream, you can pour the hand cream into a small jar and leave to cool. If you notice afterwards that the consistency is not yet optimal, you can reheat the cream and add some oil or cocoa butter and of course you can also go wild with the essential oils and choose different fragrances as desired.

Solid hand cream for the handbag

Ingredients:
- ♥ 7 g beeswax
- ♥ 30 g cocoa butter or shea butter
- ♥ 3 tsp olive oil
- ♥ 2-3 pots essential oil
- ♥ an ice cube mould or praline moulds

In fact, there is also solid hand cream that is super portionable and perfect for on the go. It may sound a bit complicated and abstract at first, but this hand cream also requires only a few ingredients and hardly any effort to make.

Step one is again to heat the cocoa butter and beeswax in a water bath or in the microwave, before you can then stir in the olive oil and the essential oil or a few spices. Stir everything together with a small whisk until the mixture is nice and even and has cooled down a bit. You can then pour the finished cream into small ice cube or praline moulds and leave to harden completely. Before that, you can also add some decoration and stir in a few dry flower petals, a few pieces of lemon peel or similar.

You can keep the finished hand cream in an air-sealed jar for several months and always take out a new cube when the last cube is slowly running out. The application is similar to liquid hand creams and you can simply run the cube over your hands a few times and then rub everything in nicely. But the practical thing is that no greasy film forms on the skin and the cream does not take so long to be absorbed, which means you can touch everything again without any problems immediately afterwards.

9. Self-tanner

Self-tanners can also be made easily and with just a few ingredients, and it doesn't always have to be the bought tanner from the drugstore, which may not suit the skin tone anyway or is too strong/weak. What's more, the homemade tanner comes without additives and with all-natural ingredients.

<u>The perfect tan through tea</u>

Ingredients:
♥   4 bags black tea
♥   100 ml lanolin
♥   100 ml sesame oil

For the simple tea tanner, you only need three ingredients, all of which you can get in a well-stocked drugstore, pharmacy or online. Lanolin - also known as wool wax - is a well-tolerated natural product that is very similar to the skin's greasy film. This is why it is often used as a base for creams and ointments, and because of its additional binding capacity of fat and water, it also supports the emulsion of the creams.

To make the self-tanner, you first need to pour 200ml of boiling water over the tea bags and let them steep for about 40 minutes so that the colour from the tea also binds well in the water. When the tea is ready and well cooled, you can add the remaining ingredients and mix well. Depending on your skin type, you can also use a little less or more tea bags and it is also possible to dilute the boiled tea with more water after it has steeped. However, you must make sure that you also adjust the other ingredients accordingly, otherwise you will have too much water and the mixture will no longer be beautiful. When everything is ready, you can put the tanner on the skin and rub it in evenly. You can put the rest in a sealable jar and store it in the fridge. Do not exceed a storage period of about one month, as the colour will fade over time.

Self-tanner with henna and black tea

Ingredients:
- ♥ 6 bags black tea
- ♥ 3 tablespoons henna powder (copper)
- ♥ 6 tablespoons coconut oil

For a self-tanning mask that you can wash off again with lukewarm water after the application time, a mixture of black tea and henna is excellent and is similarly quick to make as the first recipe.

Pour 200 ml of hot water over the six tea bags and let the tea steep for about 40 minutes. Add the henna powder in the colour copper at the beginning, but you can also adjust the colour according to your skin tone. When the tea with the powder has cooled down, you can add the six tablespoons of melted coconut oil, pour everything into a jar with a lid and let it cool down again.

This self-tanner is also ready, and you can apply the cream well on the skin, let it absorb for about 15 minutes and then rinse it off with lukewarm water. The colour will transfer to your skin a little in the meantime, so it's also very important that you slather on evenly and don't leave any big gaps. It is best to try the cream first on an area where it is not so noticeable, and you can try out the shade.

Self-tanner for spraying

Ingredients:
- ♥ A pinch of erythrulose
- ♥ 1 tablespoon aloe vera juice

If you prefer to have a spray-on self-tanner, then this recipe may be right for you. Self-tanners with erythrulose are particularly skin-friendly, as this substance has no drying properties, and it moisturises rather than takes away moisture.

To make the spray, just mix the two ingredients together well and then add more water until you have the desired strength. You can also try the tanner a few times and only then add more water or more erythrulose. However, this tanner does not work from now on, but only about three days after spraying you will see a result. So, when you first try it, make sure that you don't spray too much right away, but carefully approach the right amount.

Self-tanner with chocolate

Ingredients:
- ♥ 1 cup conventional body lotion
- ♥ 1/4 cup cocoa powder

Actually, anything with the word chocolate in its name is already good from the start, and with a little cocoa, this recipe is also convincing as an effective and, above all, good-smelling self-tanner. The two ingredients make it uncomplicated and spontaneous to make and you can replenish at any time.

Simply mix the body lotion, which you can of course also make yourself, with cocoa or some melted chocolate and mix everything evenly. After showering, you can then apply the finished cream and let it soak in for about 45 minutes. The cocoa powder has made the body lotion a little firmer, so it is no longer fully absorbed. After this time, you can rinse off the remains with lukewarm water and dry yourself off carefully. You should definitely not rub too hard, otherwise the tanning effect will no longer be on the skin, but on the towel.

10. Nail oil

There are also some remedies for dry and brittle nails and since hand creams often leave out nail care, there are extra sprays or oils for nail care.

Oil from avocado oil and tea tree oil

Ingredients:
- ♥ 80ml avocado oil
- ♥ 50 drops tea tree oil

Nail oil is comparatively easy to make, because you only need two ingredients for the basic recipe. You have to mix both ingredients vigorously and then put them into a tightly sealable bottle that is best darkened a little. With simple glass bottles, there is a risk that the oil will be destroyed by light and thus also lose its nourishing effect.

To apply the oil, you can use a small brush to spread a few drops on each nail. Then gently massage the nail oil into the nail and the nail bed and leave it to soak in. Before you use the oil the next time, you should shake the bottle again vigorously, as it is possible that avocado oil and tea tree oil separate from each other over time.

Luxury Oil for Experienced

> **Ingredients:**
> - ♥ 50 ml jojoba oil
> - ♥ 4 drops sandalwood oil
> - ♥ 4 drops cypress oil
> - ♥ 4 drops lavender oil

This oil is a little more time-consuming to prepare, but it has an even better effect, and your nails will be even better cared for. You can find the ingredients either in a pharmacy or in a well-stocked drugstore; of course, you can also order the oils on the internet.

To prepare the oil, first put the jojoba oil in a water bath and heat it carefully. The oil should only be lukewarm, so keep checking the temperature so that it does not get too hot. Once the oil has reached the right temperature, you can add the remaining ingredients and stir vigorously with a spoon or small whisk until a uniform mixture is formed. You can then pour the finished oil into a sealable jar, preferably with a slightly wider opening. This oil is not applied drop by drop to the nails and massaged in, but you leave your fingertips in it for about 10 minutes and let the oil soak in. Afterwards, however, do not wash your hands directly, but only dab the oil residues lightly with a towel so that the oil can still be absorbed.

Nail oil cream

Of course, nail care is not only available as oil, but also in cream form, which is great for your handbag. The production is just as uncomplicated and if you want, you can also refine the cream with different essential oils.

Ingredients:
- ♥ 25 ml jojoba oil
- ♥ 15 ml castor oil
- ♥ 15 ml avocado oil
- ♥ 15 ml Vaseline cream base

Simply put all the ingredients together in a water bath and heat it on a low heat until the Vaseline has become completely liquid. Then you just have to mix everything vigorously and pour it into a dark, sealable jar. After the cream has cooled down a little and become solid again, you can already use it, not only on your nails, but also on your hands.

The cream is best stored in the fridge, because it stays nice and firm there, and also lasts longer than in the bathroom cabinet.

11. Nail varnish

Nail polish is often very expensive and in the end half of it is always left dried out because the colour wasn't so nice, or you simply couldn't use it all up so quickly. But luckily there are also many recipes for beautiful nail polish and actually making it is not that difficult. And another tip, dried-up nail polish can easily be made liquid again by adding a little nail polish remover as needed and stirring everything together with a toothpick or something similar.

The basic recipe for clear lacquer

Ingredients:
- ♥ 50 ml ethanol
- ♥ 10 g benzoin (powdered resin)
- ♥ 1 g silicic acid
- ♥ 1 empty nail varnish bottle

As a base for the homemade nail polish in colour, you can either buy the necessary clear nail polish or you can also quickly make this yourself with a few ingredients. However, as the ingredients are a little more specialised this time, you may have to order some of them on the internet or you may have to do a bit of searching first.

When you have all the ingredients together, you can slowly heat the ethanol in a water bath until it is not quite boiling. Then take the pot off the heat and stir in the benzoin until it is completely dissolved and well distributed. Finally, just stir in the silica and pour everything into an empty nail polish bottle. If you are not yet completely satisfied with the result, you can experiment a little with the composition or you can opt for a purchased clear nail polish after all and just add the colour itself.

<u>Colourful nail varnish</u>

Ingredients:
- ♥ Clear lacquer
- ♥ Colour pigments

Of course, just clear nail polish is a bit boring and a polish in a nice colour looks much better on the nails. In addition to the homemade or purchased clear nail polish, all you need are a few colour pigments in the desired colour and preferably a small mortar to make them a little smaller. The finer the pigments are, the easier they are to spread with clear nail polish and the result on the nails will be much more beautiful. However, be a little careful with the amount you use and feel your way slowly to the desired shade. Often, the lacquer looks different in the bottle than it does on the nail at the end, so it is best to do a small test in between.

To make the colourful nail varnish, it is best to put the clear varnish in a small bowl. This way you can stir the colour pigments more easily and also make sure that everything actually dissolves. It is important that the colour is distributed everywhere and that the pigments have dissolved well, which may take a little time, but you will have a beautiful result to show for it. Once everything has been mixed, you can pour the polish back into an empty nail polish jar and use it directly for the next polish application.

Instead of buying extra colour pigments, you can also sustainably use old eye shadow in the desired colour and grind it into a fine powder with a mortar or a small spoon. The remaining steps are identical, and the homemade and particularly inexpensive nail varnish is ready.

Matte lacquer

Ingredients:
- ♥ 1 nail varnish of choice
- ♥ 1/2 tsp cornflour
- ♥ 1 tablespoon nail polish remover

If you prefer to wear matt nail polish, you can easily make it yourself with a little cornflour and nail polish remover. Just add a little cornflour to the coloured nail polish and mix it with nail polish remover.

Again, try it out and if the result is too dry or runny, you can simply add a little more cornflour or nail polish remover. The amount given is for a whole bottle, although the amount varies depending on the brand of nail polish. It is best to add only a small amount at first and slowly work your way up to the right consistency.

You can always test the nail polish in between and see if you are satisfied with the result.

12. Shower gel

Among cosmetic products, shower gel and shampoo are certainly the products that contain the most microplastics and also generate the most packaging waste. It's often not your fault that you have so much shower gel in your bathroom, because it's a popular gift and all too often there is some that you don't even want to use because of the smell. So why not try the more sustainable and vegan option and make your own shower gel with the desired scent?

Basic recipe

Ingredients:
- ♥ 50-60 gram natural soap
- ♥ 400 ml liquid (water or herbal tea)
- ♥ Optional: 2 tbsp vegetable oil
- ♥ Optional: 1 tsp thickener such as corn starch
- ♥ Optional: 5-10 drops of essential oils

The basic recipe for your own shower gel is very simple. You can mix it with a wide variety of essential oils or teas.
First grate the natural soap with a grater or cut it into small pieces with a knife.
At the same time, bring the water to the boil in a small pot and add either herbal or fruit tea. When the tea has finished brewing, you can bring the water to the boil again and stir in the grated soap. Stir this mixture until the soap has melted completely and everything is well mixed.

Before you add the corn starch, you can add some vegetable oil for care and a few drops of essential oil. Finally, the corn starch serves as a thickener and to prevent lumps from forming, it is best to mix it separately in a small glass and only add it to the shower gel afterwards. Be careful with the corn starch that even a very small amount is enough and too much starch will result in you getting more of a shower jelly than a shower gel. Of course, this is not a problem either, but not the desired result.

To store it, you can use old shower gel packaging that you wash out with a little hot water beforehand. This makes your shower gel even more sustainable, and you don't have to buy extra packaging. Small bottles are also good and old smoothie bottles or bottles of oils are particularly suitable for gifts.

<u>Solid shower gel</u>

Ingredients:
- ♥ 100 g cocoa butter or shea butter
- ♥ 100 g cornflour
- ♥ 100 g of the vegetable surfactant

If you prefer something in soap form instead of shower gel, you can also easily make the so-called "shower bars" yourself.

To do this, weigh the dry ingredients all into a bowl while the cocoa butter becomes liquid in a water bath. You can then add the liquid butter to the bowl and mix everything together until the dry ingredients have completely dissolved and a smooth cream has been created.

Now you can add essential oils, lemon zest, coffee powder or similar things to create the perfect smell. When everything is mixed and you are happy with the result, you can put the mixture into a silicone mould, ice cube mould or similar and leave it to cool in the fridge for a few hours. Finally, all you have to do is turn everything out of the mould and put it in a small sealable tin for storage, leaving only one cube in the shower at a time.

13. Bath bombs

The best-known and probably most popular cosmetic product to make yourself is the bath bomb, for which there are now an incredible number of different recipes. Although you need a few different ingredients and a little patience, the result is all the more beautiful and you can be creative in your choice of colours and fragrances.

Simple basic recipe

Ingredients:
- ♥ 200 gr. Baking soda
- ♥ 100 gr. citric acid
- ♥ 100 ml olive oil
- ♥ 50 gr. cornflour
- ♥ 7 drops fragrance oil
- ♥ Food colouring

The classic recipe for bubbling bath bombs is based on bicarbonate of soda and citric acid, which creates the bubbling effect when the bath bomb and water meet. The olive oil is mainly a binder and also ensures that the bath bombs nourish and moisturise the skin.

To make the beautiful balls, you first need to mix all the dry ingredients together in a bowl and add the olive oil and fragrance oil. You can then mix the whole thing well with your hands and blend it into a compact dough. You can either add the food colouring to the whole dough or divide it into a few bowls beforehand and add different colours. Just a few drops of the colour are enough, and you should be quick when mixing it in, as the liquid colour already reacts with the citric acid and the baking soda.

When the "dough" is ready, it's time to shape the balls and if you don't want to buy a bath bomb mould, you can also use small cake moulds or jars. You just have to make sure that you get the finished bath bomb out of the mould. For the classic mould, fill both halves slightly over the rim with the mixture and then press both sides well together. Leave the ball in the mould for a short time so that the halves can join together, and everything does not fall apart again straight away. After five to ten minutes, you can carefully remove the bath bomb from the mould and place it on a plate to set in the fridge for a few more hours, but preferably overnight. If you have chosen an intense fragrance, it is best to put the bath bombs in a sealable box so that your whole fridge doesn't smell of lavender or something. With the classic shapes, the dough is enough for about three bath bombs, but you can also make smaller ones or mix the amount of dough with different essential oils.

Bath salts

Ingredients:
- ♥ 1 cup sea salt (coarse-grained)
- ♥ 15 - 20 drops of essential oils (e.g. lavender oil, orange oil, rose geranium oil)
- ♥ Flower petals (e.g. lavender flowers, orange peel, rose buds)
- ♥ Glass vessel

Instead of bath bombs, you can also make bath salts super simply and you need even fewer ingredients for this. The basis for this is not sodium bicarbonate and citric acid, but coarse-grained sea salt, which can be mixed with essential oils, spices or orange peel. You are again completely free to choose the fragrance, whereby each fragrance has a different effect. Lavender baths have a very relaxing effect and are just the thing after a tiring day. Orange oil, on the other hand, has a more mood-lifting effect and rose scent is good for becoming more balanced again.

As an additive for softer skin, you can also add some odourless oil to the bath salts. You can either mix this directly into the salt or add it to a small bowl together with a portion of bath salt shortly before bathing and mix well. The second option is better for storing the salt. Even after a year, you can be sure that you can still use the pure salt mixture without any problems.

Here are a few recipe tips for baths with a special effect. Simply add the appropriate ingredients to the basic recipe and enjoy a soothing bath.

>

> The mixture of eucalyptus and peppermint has a relieving effect on colds or blocked airways. If you add five drops of eucalyptus oil and ten drops of peppermint oil to your bath salts, you will get the perfect mixture. Instead of peppermint oil, you can also use dried or fresh peppermint, although this should always be picked directly before bathing.

> Add lemon peel and a few dried needles of rosemary or some rosemary oil to your bath salts for a liberating and refreshing effect. This combination has a calming effect and even after a stressful and nerve-racking day, you can use it to calm down again.

> Ten drops of arnica oil and ten drops of spruce oil help especially with muscle and joint pain and also loosen sore muscles or cramps. After a strenuous workout, such a spruce-anica bath is just the right thing, maybe you will even avoid an impending muscle ache.

> Last but not least, the invigorating bath with three cloves, orange peel and five pots of cedar oil is a must. In case of listlessness, tiredness or similar, this bath helps to get going again with more energy and to cope with the daily tasks.

Ingredients:
- ♥ 250 ml extra virgin olive oil
- ♥ Two handfuls of fresh petals
- ♥ 10 drops of the appropriate essential fragrance oil

For a soothing bath oil, you can collect a few flower petals or fresh herbs in summer and pour a cold-pressed oil over them. After only two to three weeks, the leaves will have transferred their scent to the oil and, depending on your needs, you can also add some essential oil afterwards to make the oil smell even more intense. Spices such as cloves, cinnamon sticks or pieces of orange and lemon peel also look good in the bath oil. A mixture of olive oil, honey and a little milk is especially good for your skin.

Foam bath

Bubble baths are a very special bathing experience and there is hardly anyone who likes to bathe without a nice portion of foam. Since bath bombs bubble up especially at the beginning but stop again after a while and leave only a little foam behind, there are also extra recipes for bubble baths.

Ingredients:
- ♥ Neutral liquid soap
- ♥ 20 ml almond oil
- ♥ Fragrance oil
- ♥ Soap colouring or food colouring
- ♥ optionally a spoonful of honey

To make the liquid bath additive, all you have to do is mix some neutral liquid soap with 20 ml of almond oil and then add a fragrance oil of your choice. For a beautiful colour, you can stir in a few drops of soap or food colouring, whereby even a small amount can lead to an intense result. For a special caring experience, you can add a teaspoon of honey and stir it into the whole mixture. If you don't have liquid honey on hand, you can also carefully heat a little more solid honey in the microwave or in a water bath until it is liquid enough.

14. Lipstick

There are generally two differences when making lipsticks. You can either make a nourishing lip balm or a lipstick with colour. Of course, you can also combine both options and add a few colour pigments to the lip balm.

A small tip for more sustainability: If you have lipstick residue, you can carefully melt it over a candle, in the microwave or in a water bath and put it into a new jar. It's best not to choose the typical screw-on lipstick packaging for this, but a small cream jar from which you can apply the lipstick with your finger. You can use this method especially for leftover lip balm, but it also works well for coloured lipsticks and even if the sticks have slightly different shades, you will get a nice new mixture out of it.

Ingredients:
- ♥ 15 g jojoba oil
- ♥ 15 g almond oil
- ♥ 5 g beeswax
- ♥ Teaspoon honey

Nourishing lip balm with honey

A nourishing balm with honey is not only easy to make, but also particularly effective and provides a lot of moisture for dry lips.

To make the lip care, put the oils together with the beeswax in a small bowl and then heat it in a water bath. You can stir a little at a time, and when everything has mixed well, you can add the honey at the end. The choice of honey doesn't really matter, and you can also choose a slightly firmer honey, as it will become liquid in the water bath anyway. You can then put the finished lip balm directly into a small container and leave it to cool until it has completely set. The honey also gives the balm an antibacterial effect. If you have very irritated lips, it may sting a little when you apply the care. However, this is not a bad sign, but only shows that it is starting to work and is fighting against the bacteria.

Vegan Lip Balm with Vanilla Flavouring

Ingredients:
- ♥ 8 g beeswax substitute
- ♥ 20 g coconut oil
- ♥ 20 g shea butter
- ♥ 4 drops vanilla flavouring

As a vegan alternative to the lip balm with honey, you can also try this lip balm based on coconut oil and shea butter. To make it, put all the ingredients in a water bath and melt them over medium heat. Instead of the beeswax, you can also use a little more shea butter, or you can ask your drugstore for sensible alternatives. When everything has melted, you can add the pith of half a vanilla bean in addition to the vanilla flavouring, or some cinnamon if you prefer something more Christmassy. The cinnamon also has a similar antibacterial effect as the honey and thus prevents inflammation in chapped areas. As before, you can then divide the finished balm into a few cream jars and let it cool until it has set.

15. Healing ointments

Lavender ointment for calming

Ingredients:
- ♥ 100 ml lavender oil
- ♥ 10 g beeswax

A very simple ointment with a wide range of effects is this lavender ointment, for which you first need only two ingredients. Put the oil together with the beeswax in a bowl and slowly melt the beeswax in a water bath. Keep stirring with a small spoon so that the mixture is even. When everything has mixed nicely, you can check the consistency with a small amount on a spoon and see if the ointment is too solid or too liquid. If necessary, you can add a little more oil or beeswax before filling and if the lavender scent is still too weak for you, you can also mix in a few drops of essential oil.

The finished ointment is best stored in small ointment jars or a jar with a screw cap so that it does not dry out and has a longer shelf life. It is also best to store the jars in a cool place protected from light and use the ointment within the next six months.

Lavender oil has a pleasant calming effect and also has an anti-inflammatory and pain-relieving effect and helps with dry skin. This ointment is therefore a real all-rounder and is especially good in the wintertime. If you have problems falling asleep, you can also rub some of the lavender ointment on your hands or under your nose and you will see that you can sleep much faster and better.

Ingredients:
- ♥ fresh ribwort leaves
- ♥ Olive oil
- ♥ optional coconut oil
- ♥ Beeswax

Finding a really good ointment against itchy insect bites is not that easy and most of the time the ointments from the drugstore or pharmacy only work for a short time or smell unpleasant. However, so that you are not so plagued by annoying mosquito bites in summer, you can get to work with a little ribwort, olive oil and beeswax to make your own ointment against itching.

To make the actual ointment, you first need to process ribwort plantain and olive oil together to make an oil, although this is not too difficult. You can determine the amount of oil and leaves yourself, depending on the desired amount and intensity of the ointment. The best amount is about six to eight larger leaves of ribwort plantain per 100 ml of olive oil. These should be as dry and clean as possible so that the oil becomes clear. The leaves must then be cut into small pieces before you put them into a jar with the oil. If you also want to add some coconut oil for a particularly moisturising ointment, you should replace about 20% of the olive oil with already liquefied coconut oil and add it to the leaves. The finished mixture must now infuse for about two weeks and be shaken a little every day so that the substances from the ribwort plantain are well distributed in the oil. After this time, you only have to pour the oil through a sieve and the homemade ribwort oil is ready.

To make the ointment, you will then need some beeswax, whereby you can calculate with about 12 g per 100 ml of oil. If you prefer a creamier ointment, simply omit two or three grams and if you want it to be more of a solid ointment, you can also add more beeswax. To make the ointment, simply follow the same steps as for the lavender ointment and heat all the ingredients in a water bath before pouring the mixture into small jars and storing them in a cool, dark place.

For insect bites, you can then apply the ointment directly to the sting and massage it in gently with circular movements. You can repeat the treatment up to four times a day and the ribwort ointment also has a soothing effect on wasp or bee stings.

Red clover ointment against dry skin

Ingredients:
- ♥ 100 ml red clover plant oil extract
- ♥ 5 g beeswax
- ♥ 10 g lanolin
- ♥ essential oil

With this ointment, too, you can produce the red clover oil yourself if you have some time. For the specified amount of 100 ml, you only need to mix 100 ml of olive oil with the flowers and leaves of red clover. Leave this mixture in a cool place for about two weeks, stirring daily, and wait until the aroma and active ingredients of the clover have transferred to the oil. After the two weeks, you can pour the finished oil through a sieve and either fill it into small bottles or use it directly to make the skin balm.

To finish the ointment, you only need to heat beeswax and lanolin in a water bath and add them to the finished oil. Since clover is rather odourless, you can also add an essential oil of your choice.

The substances in the red clover, which dissolve in the oil during the time, ensure that the water storage capacity in the cells increases and thus the moisture is retained better over a longer period of time. In addition, the ointment also works against wrinkles and makes the skin look firmer and younger. With this ointment, you not only have a good hand cream, but also a cheap and effective anti-ageing product.

Cold balm

Ingredients:
♥ 50 ml vegetable oil
♥ 5 g beeswax
♥ 6-8 drops essential oil

To make an effective balm against colds, you don't need many ingredients and depending on which essential oil you choose, you have a different range of action.

The preparation is very quick and uncomplicated and already after you have heated the oil together with the beeswax in a water bath, you can add the essential oils of your choice, stir everything and fill it into a suitable jar. If you choose herbal oils such as peppermint, sage or rosemary, you can also mix the 50 ml of vegetable oil with a handful of herbs two weeks earlier instead of the essential oil, let everything infuse and pour it off before processing it into an ointment. This way you don't have to buy an essential oil and you also work more sustainably.

Chestnut ointment against heavy legs and inflammations

Ingredients:
- ♥ 30 ml horse chestnut tincture
- ♥ 30 ml olive oil
- ♥ 15 g lanolin
- ♥ 4 g beeswax

This particular ointment is a little more complicated to make and especially if you decide to make the chestnut tincture yourself as well, you will need to allow a little more time.

To make the tincture from horse chestnuts, you need horse chestnuts and 40 % alcohol by volume to pour on, in addition to the ingredients listed. The amount of both is variable depending on the amount of product you want. You should have about enough chestnuts to half-fill the storage jar when cut into small pieces. In the first step, you need to cut the horse chestnuts roughly into quarters and optionally remove the skin before chopping everything further with a blender. The small pieces then go into a glass jar, which should ideally be darkened so that the tincture is not destroyed by UV radiation. Now you have to add the neutral alcohol until the chestnuts are completely covered. After about four to six weeks of infusion, you can pour the finished tincture through a coffee or tea filter and squeeze out the residue from the chestnuts again so that as little liquid as possible remains in the horse chestnuts.

With the finished tincture, you can then make the ointment directly, as with the other recipes, by putting the tincture with the olive oil and the two solid ingredients in a water bath and letting it melt. Optionally, you can also add some essential oil of juniper berries or cypress, which will enhance the effect even more. Fill it into a salve jar and wait until the chestnut salve is solid and you can smear it on your arms and legs to relieve pain and improve blood flow.

16. Toothpaste

Even if it seems a bit abstract at first and you can't imagine that you can also easily make cosmetic items for dental care yourself, you can actually find some good recipes here to make sustainable and effective toothpastes.

Basic recipe for toothpaste

Ingredients:
- ♥ 5 tbsp. coconut oil
- ♥ 3 tsp bicarbonate of soda
- ♥ 1 pinch xylitol
- ♥ 1 pinch turmeric
- ♥ 1 tsp peppermint oil

For a toothpaste made from natural ingredients, which is even vegan, you only need a few ingredients. You probably already have many of them in your kitchen. Before you start making your own toothpaste, however, you should be aware that it will be a big change, especially in terms of taste, and you may need a few days to get used to the new cream. To avoid having to throw away large quantities, try only a small portion at first and see if you want to use a little more peppermint oil or add other flavourings.

As with most homemade cosmetic recipes, this preparation is very simple. After you have melted the coconut oil in a water bath, you can stir in the baking soda. Once you have mixed everything together, add the rest of the ingredients and pour the finished mixture into a jar or cream tube to cool.

When brushing your teeth, simply apply a small amount of the cream to your toothbrush as usual and brush your teeth as normal. The cleaning effect is the same as that of a normal toothpaste you can buy, and the all-natural ingredients make it even better for your teeth and gums. You can also start by using the new toothpaste only every other time and let your teeth get used to the change to an all-natural product.

Mouthwash

Ingredients:
- ♥ 250 ml hydrolate or distilled water
- ♥ 1 tablespoon bicarbonate of soda
- ♥ 1 tbsp xylitol
- ♥ 10 drops essential oils

Also, for those who like to take extra care of their teeth with mouthwash, there are some super simple recipes and since the ingredients are similar to toothpaste, you don't even have to buy extra stuff.

Simply put all the ingredients listed into a small glass bottle, stir everything vigorously or shake the contents a few times and you have your ready-made sustainable mouthwash. The essential oils mainly serve as flavour carriers in this recipe. You can of course adjust the number of drops depending on how intense you want the mouthwash to be.

Small ingredient profile:
Since toothpaste is particularly important for a functioning effect, you will find all the individual ingredients with their effect briefly explained here once again and can thus understand that even a few ingredients are actually enough to carefully care for your teeth.

Baking soda: As a natural mineral salt, baking soda stimulates saliva production in the mouth and thus ensures that the self-cleaning process in the mouth gets going again. It also has an antibacterial effect and prevents tooth decay and tartar formation. For addition to toothpaste, the sodium bicarbonate should be ground as finely as possible and, if necessary, you can also briefly put it in the mortar again before stirring it in.

Coconut oil: This oil also has an antibacterial effect and inhibits the growth of bacteria in the oral cavity. In addition, it also has a soothing effect on the gums and quickly reduces swelling and inflammation.

Xylitol: At first you may wonder what sugar has to do in a toothpaste, but in fact the well-known birch sugar has a supporting effect and, unlike normal household sugar, reduces bacterial growth. In addition, xylitol also helps to re-mineralise the teeth and thus ensures stronger and more resistant teeth.

Essential oils: Most oils that are suitable for making toothpaste have a strong antibacterial effect, are antiviral and anti-inflammatory. Of course, taste also plays an important role here, because everyone probably prefers brushing their teeth with a good-tasting toothpaste than with a nasty one.

17. Perfume

Perhaps you already have the perfect fragrance in mind for your own personal perfume, or you want to switch to a more sustainable and, above all, chemical-free option. The perfumes that are currently available for purchase actually all have a very long list of ingredients made up of some complex terms. Many products also use animal testing to test skin compatibility. For your own perfume, you don't need all these things and can decide for yourself which ingredients you would like to have in your perfume, which combination of scents you want or how much you want to make. Besides the typical perfume for spraying, there is even solid perfume that you can apply similar to a body cream.

Lavender perfume

Ingredients:
- ♥ 10 ml ethanol
- ♥ 10 drops lavender
- ♥ 10 drops lemon
- ♥ 3 drops vanilla

To make perfume, you first need a carrier, such as ethanol, which absorbs the fragrances and also serves as a diluent. The pure essential oils usually have a very intense smell, and it is best to dilute them a little before applying.

To make the lavender perfume, you need a few essential oils in the scent of lavender, lemon and vanilla in addition to the ethanol. This combination takes away some of the intensity of the lavender and the perfume will not be quite so intrusive.

Simply mix the alcohol with the different oils and put everything together in a spray bottle. Leave the bottle to infuse for two to three weeks so that the fragrance molecules can disperse well, and the perfume has a generally uniform scent. During the waiting time, you can also shake the perfume gently from time to time to mix the ingredients even better.

If you want to use more natural products, you can also mix some fresh lavender flowers into the ethanol and let them infuse for a few weeks. You may have to wait a little longer to achieve the desired intensity, but the perfume will smell more natural. After the infusion time, you should still pour the mixture through a fine sieve or coffee filter so that you can separate the flowers from the finished perfume. If you leave the blossoms in for too long, the scent may either become too intense or the mixture may collapse and no longer smell good at all.

Ingredients:
- ♥ essential oils
- ♥ 10g persimmon butter
- ♥ 20g jojoba oil
- ♥ 4-5g beeswax

Solid perfume

The solid perfume does not need a carrier such as ethanol. Besides the essential oil, you only need cocoa butter, jojoba oil and beeswax for the production.

To make it, you can slowly melt the cocoa butter together with the oil and beeswax in a water bath. When you have mixed everything well and a nice uniform mixture has formed, you can add a few essential oils and fill the perfume into ice cube moulds, cream tubes or similar. Now leave it to harden in a dark and cool place and then put it in airtight tins. For application, you can then take out a cube or simply pick up some solid perfume directly from the jar with your fingers and spread it on the desired areas. However, do not rub too hard and first try out how much you need so that a pleasant fragrance surrounds you.

<u>Rose perfume without ethanol</u>

Ingredients:
- ♥ 10 ml jojoba oil
- ♥ 20 drops rose oil
- ♥ 10 drops sandalwood oil

If you are looking for a perfume to spray but which can be made without ethanol, you can try this recipe. In addition to the suggested combination of essential oils, you can of course also opt for other fragrances and refine the jojoba oil according to your own wishes. It is made according to the same principle as lavender oil and you can simply put all the ingredients into a sealable bottle. Leave it in a cool place for about two weeks, stirring it a little every two days so that the fragrance molecules are evenly distributed. You can also add a few fresh rose petals to the mixture, but then you should use a few drops less of the essential rose oil.

After the mixture is ready, you can use the perfume directly and store it in a cool place with little light. With this perfume, however, you must be aware that it may leave stains on clothing due to the oil content. This is not a problem with ethanol-based perfumes, but before you mess up your top with oil stains that are difficult to remove, it is best to only use oil-based perfumes directly on the skin.

18. Deo

Deodorant accompanies you in your daily life and all too often there are discussions about how sustainable the products from the drugstores actually are and whether roll-on or spray-on deodorants are better. So that you can use deodorant in future without a guilty conscience, here are a few simple recipes to make yourself. No matter whether you prefer spray deodorants, roll-on deodorants or deodorant cream, you can make everything yourself with just a few ingredients and you certainly have everything you need for most recipes at home.

Deodorant cream

To combine the deodorant with a caring effect, you can also make a deodorant cream instead of liquid deodorant, which is just as effective against annoying perspiration odour.

Ingredients:
- ♥ 30 g coconut oil
- ♥ 15 g baking soda
- ♥ 15 g starch
- ♥ Essential oil

With just four ingredients and ten minutes of time, you have the finished result in your jar and no longer have to worry about your deodorant failing. Melt the coconut oil again in a water bath and stir in the baking soda and cornflour. It may take a little longer for both products to dissolve completely and if the cream becomes too thick, you can also add some more coconut oil. Finally, you only need a little essential oil of your choice and when you have stirred this in, you can pour the cream into a small jar, which is always good to take with you on the go.

The mixture of sodium bicarbonate and starch not only works against the smell of sweat, it also has an antibacterial effect. If you want, you can also apply the cream to your arms and legs. The essential oils also mask possible perspiration odours, so you are doubly protected. However, it is best to apply the cream before you put on a top so that it can be absorbed well and not everything sticks to your clothes.

Sustainable Roll-on

Ingredients:
- ♥ 100 ml tap water
- ♥ 12 g (1 tbsp) cornflour
- ♥ 12 g (1 tbsp) baking soda

For your own roll deodorant, you need even fewer ingredients and you should already have all the necessary utensils in your kitchen cupboard. In addition to the ingredients for the deodorant, however, you also need an empty roll deodorant jar into which you can pour your finished mixture.

First boil the tap water and then let it cool down again to about 50 degrees. Now you can add the cornflour and the bicarbonate of soda and mix everything with a small whisk until a uniform liquid has formed. You can also add essential oils to this deodorant, but even without them it works well against the smell of sweat and is not overpowering.

When everything is ready, you can put the deodorant in the appropriate glass bottle, but let it finish cooling before using it. If you no longer have an empty bottle at home, you can also buy one or ask friends if anyone has one to spare. These bottles are very expensive to produce and comparatively material-intensive, so every reused bottle is a gain.

Spray deodorant with a hint of lime

Ingredients:
- ♥ 50 ml tap water
- ♥ 1 tsp bicarbonate of soda
- ♥ 5 drops lime oil
- ♥ 2 drops tea tree oil

Spray deodorants come in a wide range of variations and you too can get creative when you make your own deodorant. The use of different fragrances brings variety and so you even have deodorant and perfume in one product.

Spray deodorants are also easy to make. After you have boiled the tap water, you can stir in the baking soda and add the essential oils a short time later. The lime oil adds freshness, and the tea tree oil has an additional antibacterial effect. When you have mixed everything together well, you can put the liquid in a small spray bottle and store it in a cool place. It is possible that the bicarbonate of soda will separate from the water again somewhat over time, but you can usually avoid this by shaking it regularly before use. If the separation still occurs, you can heat the mixture slowly in a water bath and stir it again and again until a nice mixture has formed.

Spray deodorant with fresh elderberry

Ingredients:
- ♥ 1 elderflower umbel
- ♥ ½ organic lemon zest
- ♥ 100 ml water
- ♥ 1 tsp bicarbonate of soda

Fresh elderberries have an incredibly intense scent and also make a good composition in deodorant. The scent is reminiscent of summer and freshness and thus easily masks the smell of sweat.

To make this deodorant, first remove the flowers from the umbel and put them together with the lemon peel into a sealable glass. Now add the boiled water to this glass, but it should no longer be too hot. It is best to wait about five minutes after boiling and only then add it. Place the mixture in the refrigerator overnight so that the elderflowers can release their fragrance, and everything can infuse a little. The next day, you can pour the liquid through a sieve or a fine filter so that you only have the water in a glass at the end. Add the bicarbonate of soda to the water and stir vigorously so that the bicarbonate of soda dissolves well. This recipe is also ready! You can put the deodorant back into a small spray bottle and store it in a cool place. Because of the small quantities, you should not have a problem using up the deodorant before it is no longer as effective, but if you do have some left over, you should pour it out after about a year and make a new deodorant.

DIY hair products

1. Shampoo

Of course, you can not only make cosmetic products for your body yourself, but hair products can also be made easily and with only a few ingredients. For example, homemade shampoo is much more environmentally friendly, and you can be sure that you have a vegan and animal-free alternative.

<u>Soap-based chamomile shampoo</u>

Ingredients:
- ♥ 25 ml camomile flower tincture
- ♥ 25 g dried chamomile flowers
- ♥ 350 ml distilled water
- ♥ 15 g scraped curd soap
- ♥ 10 drops chamomile essential oil

An easy way to make your own shampoo is to use curd or liquid soap as a base. You can refine the soap with different essential oils or dried herbs and flowers. Because it is so easy to make, you can always try out new recipes.

To make the shampoo, you first need to boil half of the distilled water, pour it over the dried flowers and let it steep for about three hours. Instead of the blossoms, you can also use two to three sachets of chamomile tea and pour this over the boiled water. After the infusion time, boil the remaining water and slowly dissolve the curd soap in it. Since it melts more quickly in small pieces, it is a good idea to grate it a little first or cut it into small pieces with a knife. While the soap is simmering, pour the chamomile water through a sieve and catch all the flowers. If the sieve is still too coarse, you can also use a coffee filter or similar so that the water is as clear as possible afterwards. Now all you have to do is mix everything together and add essential oil or camomile flower tincture as needed. For a more neutral shampoo, you can also omit these ingredients or replace them with a little more dried flowers or tea. Your shampoo is ready to fill and can be transferred into small bottles. To apply, simply put a portion the size of a chestnut on your hand, rub everything well into your hair and let it soak in for a few minutes. Then wash the shampoo again with warm water and apply a conditioner of your choice.

Ingredients:
- ♥ Juice of half a lemon
- ♥ 1 egg yolk
- ♥ 1 dash of cognac or rum

For more shine and volume, use this shampoo with egg yolk and lemon juice, which, however, does not keep that long and is best used within two weeks. Simply mix all the ingredients together well and then put them in a small jar in the fridge. For use, you can put the shampoo out of the fridge about an hour earlier so that it gets some temperature, and you can mix everything again. Depending on the size of the yolk, the amount is enough for about two hair washes. Therefore, it is not necessarily suitable as a regular shampoo, but you can always use it as a quick cure in between. In addition, make sure that you do not wash your hair too hot, otherwise the egg yolk can leave residues in the hair and, of course, lukewarm or cold water gives the hair a nicer shine and does not stress it as much.

Quick rye flour shampoo against greasy hair

Ingredients:
- ♥ 250 ml water
- ♥ 4 tbsp rye flour or wholemeal rye flour

This two-ingredient shampoo is one of those lightning recipes. When you realise that you have forgotten to buy or make new shampoo, it is the perfect emergency solution. Even so, the rye flour shampoo is good for tackling very greasy hair in particular and ensuring that your hair is not greasy the very next day.

To make it, all you have to do is put the water in a jar with the flour, screw the lid on and shake everything vigorously until you get a milky and gel-like consistency. If you are using wholemeal flour, you should let the liquid sit for about two hours so that the flour can dissolve well. To use, you can pour the necessary amount into your hair, massage the shampoo in a little and let it work for five minutes. It is no wonder that the shampoo does not foam, after all, it does not contain any soap, which is normally responsible for the foam. Nevertheless, it works very well and because of the few ingredients and the simple production, it is particularly sustainable. If you want, you can also add a few drops of an essential oil at the end so that you also have a small fragrance note in the shampoo. When making the shampoo, however, make sure that you really only use rye flour, because wheat or spelt flour has too high a gluten content, which ensures that the shampoo becomes sticky and ends up stuck in the hair in lumps.

Solid shampoo

Ingredients:
- ♥   125 g cornflour
- ♥   120 g SLSA surfactant
- ♥   60 g shea butter
- ♥   10 drops tea tree essential oil

There are also some recipes for solid shampoo and by using surfactant you can make sure that the shampoo soap also lathers properly and has a good conditioning effect.
SLSA surfactant is a very mild surfactant and therefore does not unnecessarily irritate the scalp when used. However, it is best to wear a mouth guard when making it, as it may be that the surfactant dusts a little and thus irritates your respiratory tract.

To make the shampoo, you first need to mix the starch and the surfactant together in a bowl. At the same time, you can melt the shea butter in a water bath and stir in some food colouring if you would like a colourful soap. This recipe also works with cocoa butter, but the consistency is slightly better with shea butter. Before you then add the liquid butter to the dry ingredients, you can stir in some essential oils and mix everything well again.

Together with the starch and the surfactant, the mixture should become a kneadable but not too crumbly mass, which you can put into a soap mould or silicone mould after careful kneading. Keep pressing everything down so that the shampoo becomes compact and no large air pockets form. Now you just have to let the soap harden for several hours or overnight and your homemade solid shampoo is ready.

To use, simply rub the bar of soap gently into your hair and let everything foam up nicely.

Afterwards, you can run your hands through your hair again and massage the shampoo in properly so that you also care for your scalp well.

After showering, you should rinse the shampoo off again with cool water so that the remaining foam dissolves and the soap can dry well again. Otherwise, the moisture may soak into the soap too much and soften everything again over time. It is also best to always store the shampoo in such a way that some air can get to the soap from all sides, so that it has a chance to dry well again after showering.

Essential oils against greasy hair
Peppermint
Cypress
Lemon

Essential oils against dry hair
Lavender
Cedar wood
Rosemary
Tea tree oil

Essential oils for hair growth
Peppermint
Cedar wood
Lavender
Thyme
Rosemary
Tea tree oil

Essential oils against hair loss
Sage
Incense
Rosemary
Lavender

2. Conditioner

Conditioning hair conditioners can also be made with just a few ingredients. The simplest of them even require only one or two ingredients. When it comes to conditioners, there are a few different products, and you can choose between products for washing out and "leave-in" conditioners.

<u>Simple green tea rinse</u>

Ingredients:
- ♥ Green tea
- ♥ Water

This simple hair conditioner made from green tea is uncomplicated and can be made at any time. All you have to do is add a few bags of green tea to hot water, let it steep and then pour it over your hair after washing out the shampoo. Do not wash out the tea afterwards but leave it in the hair so that it can be absorbed.

<u>Leave-in Conditioner</u>

Ingredients:
- ♥ 40 g linseed
- ♥ 400 ml tap water or distilled water
- ♥ 1-2 tbsp. hair care vegetable oil
- ♥ optionally 5 tr. essential oil

Conditioners in the form of a "leave-in" product are particularly practical, as you can simply massage them into damp hair after washing. Besides the simple green tea variant, there are many other ideas. For example, you can also make an effective conditioner against dry and damaged hair from linseed, a little water and vegetable oil.

For the rinse, first boil the water and stir in the flax seeds. Then let these swell in the hot water until a gel-like consistency has formed. When you dip a spoon into the liquid and a slightly viscous layer accumulates around it, the gel is ready, and you can pour it all off through a fine sieve. Stir some vegetable oil and a few drops of essential oil into the cooled flaxseed gel and you have a super simple, and above all, cheap conditioner. However, as this conditioner only keeps for about a week in the fridge, you shouldn't make too much at once. You can also freeze leftovers in ice cube moulds or similar so that you don't have to throw anything away and always have a suitable portion of conditioner on hand.

Instead of flaxseed gel, you can also make or buy your own aloe vera gel and use it for the conditioner. Just try both once and then decide which product has a better effect on your hair.

Solid rinse

Similar to shampoo, conditioner can also be easily made in soap form. This gives you a very space-saving option for taking both shampoo and conditioner with you on a trip.

Ingredients:
- ♥ 3 tsp shea butter
- ♥ 2 tsp beeswax
- ♥ 2 tsp cocoa butter
- ♥ 2 tsp coconut oil
- ♥ 2 tsp mango butter
- ♥ 2 tsp avocado oil

The solid conditioner is quick to make! After you have melted the butter and coconut oil in a water bath, you can add the avocado oil and essential oils of your choice. Mix everything together. If you want an extra pretty piece of conditioner, you can also add some food colouring. Now fill all the ingredients into soap moulds or silicone moulds and leave the conditioner to set overnight.

To use, you can gently pull the piece through damp hair, distributing the conditioner from the roots to the ends. You can also run your hands through your hair to make sure that the conditioner is distributed everywhere. As this recipe is not a leave-in conditioner, you will need to rinse everything out of your hair with warm water. Before you do this, you can leave the conditioner on for a few minutes so that it works properly and actually supports the hair.

3. Hair treatment

Conditioning your hair is a good thing and you should take the time to do it at least every fortnight. This will also make your hair more durable in the long run and you will have fewer problems with split ends or too dry hair.

Ingredients:
- ♥ 1 avocado
- ♥ 2 tablespoons jojoba oil or olive oil
- ♥ 1 squeeze lemon juice

Moisturising cure from avocado and olive oil

Especially for dry and straw-like hair, this treatment is a true miracle cure, and you will notice a significant improvement after just a few applications. The natural fatty acids in the avocado provide more moisture, but still do not make the hair look greasy.

To make the treatment, first mash the avocado flesh with a fork and add the olive oil. For more freshness and a longer shelf life, add a dash of lemon juice, mix everything together and you are ready to apply the treatment. Apply the treatment to dry hair, avoiding the scalp and roots. After about ten minutes, you can rinse the avocado treatment with lukewarm water and wash your hair with shampoo.

Of course, you don't have to wash your hair right away, but you can make sure that all the remnants of the treatment are out of your hair and that you don't still have a piece of avocado hanging somewhere.

Fight split ends with banana and almonds

Ingredients:
- ♥ 1 ripe banana
- ♥ 2 to 3 drops of almond oil
- ♥ a little lemon juice if necessary

This treatment is ready to apply after just a few minutes and you will feel a change after only ten minutes. Again, mash the pulp of the banana with a fork and then add the almond oil. All you have to do now is apply this mixture to your dry hair, this time you can also proceed to the roots and scalp. Massage everything in and let it soak in for a few minutes before washing the treatment out again with warm water.

Similar to the avocado cure, you should not make this cure too far in advance, but best just before using it, so that it does not go bad and you have made half for nothing. If you have some left over, you can also easily freeze the amount and sprinkle with a little lemon juice before using it again. You may find that the banana turns slightly brown as it thaws, although this is not a sign that it is nothing anymore, it is just due to the warmer temperature and air.

Rinse cure from apple cider vinegar

Ingredients:
- ♥ 1 glass of water
- ♥ 1 teaspoon apple cider vinegar
- ♥ 1 fresh lemon

To make a conditioner and cure in one, you can simply mix one part apple cider vinegar with 9 parts water, add a little lemon juice and distribute everything in the hair.

Then let this mixture dry together with your hair and let it absorb completely. Even if the apple cider vinegar smells a little intense at first, you can be reassured because as soon as your hair is dry, the smell will also be gone.

<u>Nourishing cure with egg</u>

Ingredients:
- ♥ 2 egg yolk
- ♥ 1 egg white
- ♥ Juice of one lemon
- ♥ 1 tsp honey

Not only the shampoo with egg works wonders, eggs also do well in nourishing hair treatments and provide stronger and fresher hair. The honey adds extra shine to the treatment, and you can care for your hair and scalp without any chemical additives.

To make the cure, simply mix all the ingredients in a bowl and stir the honey well into the egg. Naturally liquid honey is best here, as warmed honey may be too hot and thus cause the egg to stagnate. In addition to the scent of lemon, you can also mix in other essential oils to cover the smell of the egg, which can be more intense depending on the egg.

Before using the treatment, you should wash your hair thoroughly and rinse out all shampoo residues before massaging the treatment into the hair while it is still damp. You can do this from the roots to the tips and the scalp does not have to be left out, as the treatment does not contain any irritating substances. After about ten minutes, you can rinse out the treatment, but you should not take a shower that is too hot, otherwise the protein will start to set and small lumps may remain in the hair.

If you have some curd left over, you can store it in a tightly sealed jar in the fridge for about three days, although it should actually all be used the first time. You can also use smaller eggs or just use one large egg and then leave out the second yolk. It takes a few tries until you find the right mixture, but afterwards you will get smooth and soft hair with regular care.

4. Hair oil

If you are in a hurry and don't have time for a hair treatment, you can also do something good for your hair with hair oil and provide more moisture, more shine or less frizzy curls. You only need two or three ingredients to make many oils, and because of the oil base, a hair oil usually lasts much longer than a treatment with a similar effect.

Ingredients:
- ♥ Sesame oil or olive oil
- ♥ Tea of choice

Hair oil with fragrance

In order to not only care for your hair with an oil, but also to provide a pleasant smell at the same time, you can simply add a tea bag to a vegetable oil of your choice and let everything steep.

There is about one tea bag per quarter litre and, depending on the type of tea, you can obtain a different intensity by the infusion time or the amount of tea. With herbal teas such as peppermint, jasmine or green tea, the scent is often transferred a little faster. You can usually take the tea bag out of the oil again after four days of resting and squeeze it again so that the oil from the tea bag also ends up in the bottle. However, if you prefer to use a fruit tea or add a few cinnamon sticks, orange peel or cloves to the oil, the transfer may take a little longer and the oil may not have taken on the scent sufficiently until after about a week. To test this, you can simply smell the oil again and again in between, stir everything or spread a small sample on your hair and check whether the scent is already sufficient.

For subsequent application, take about a hazelnut-sized portion on your hand, spread it between your palms and then apply it to your hair. It is best to leave out the roots a little so that it does not look as if you have greasy hair. For shorter hair you can use a little less oil, for very long hair you need a little more. If you still have some oil on your hands at the end, you can also apply it to your arms or legs and use it as skin care.

Properly care for dry hair

Ingredients:
- ♥ 100 ml nut oil such as walnut oil or hazelnut oil
- ♥ 100 ml jojoba oil

If you are struggling with dry hair, it is often not only due to a lack of moisture, but also because your hair lacks nutrients. To make up for this lack and give your hair a fresh shine again, you can simply put a little nut oil together with jojoba oil in a bottle, shake everything and apply to your hair.

You can then either use this oil in the same way as the first oil and you only distribute a small amount into your hair, or you use it as a cure and distribute about four tablespoons of it into your freshly washed hair. Then wrap your hair in a towel before washing out the remains of the oil again with water and a little shampoo after an hour.

Anti-splitting oil

Ingredients:
- ♥ 4 tbsp argan oil
- ♥ 1 tablespoon lemon juice

There is also a perfect remedy for dry and brittle hair, and hair oil made from argan oil works particularly well. This oil contains a lot of vitamin E, which is a good remedy for brittle and dry hair. Simply mix both ingredients well together with a fork or small whisk and then spread it on your hair. If you don't want to rinse the oil out again, you should only use about half the amount, otherwise your hair may look greasy and residue from the oil may transfer to your clothes. However, if you use it as a treatment, you can massage the entire amount into your hair and then wrap it in a small towel so that the oil can be absorbed well. After a good half hour, you can rinse out the oil residue with a little shampoo and your hair will look much stronger and more beautiful again.

5. Dry shampoo

There is not always enough time to wash your hair, and in an emergency, you may have to resort to dry shampoo. The absolute emergency alternative, which is possible at any time, is simply to add a little flour to greasy hair. But depending on your hair colour and skin type, this trick is quickly noticed, and others immediately realise that there was no time to wash your hair. In the future, however, you can also combat greasy hair with natural and homemade dry shampoos that match your colour type.

Basic recipe

Ingredients:
- ♥ 2 tbsp corn or potato starch
- ♥ 1 tsp cocoa powder
- ♥ 1 tsp bicarbonate of soda
- ♥ optionally some essential oil

To make the dry shampoo, you only need two to three ingredients, depending on your hair colour, and you'll have a small emergency portion ready to go in no time. If your hair colour tends towards dark brown or black, you can use a teaspoon of cocoa to colour the starch, as in the recipe. If you have reddish hair, you can replace the cocoa with the same amount of cinnamon. The good thing about cinnamon is also that the smell in your hair goes away quickly and you don't smell intensely of cinnamon and biscuits all day when you use the dry shampoo. For blonde hair, you can omit the cocoa or cinnamon completely and just add the starch to the hair together with the baking soda. For a pleasant smell, you can also add some essential oil, although the powder may start to clump a little.

In order to use dry shampoo properly and avoid major light stains being visible in your hair, there are a few important steps you should follow when using it. After brushing your hair thoroughly, you can either stand by the bathtub or sink with your head bent forward so that your hair falls in front of your face, Now take some powder on your fingers and massage it all over, evenly like actual shampoo. When you feel you are done, you can stand back up and gently remove the remaining powder with a towel or brush. Alternatively, you can use a powder brush to carefully spread the dry shampoo all over and then massage it in a little more with your hands.

Depending on the length of your hair and how greasy it is, different application methods are suitable, and perhaps you have a personal approach. The only important thing is that you don't end up with a big spot of dry shampoo somewhere that sticks out brightly from your hair.

End

Equipped with a large number of recipes, you can now get started and go into the production of your own cosmetic products. After all, it's a much nicer feeling when you can sit in front of the TV in the evening after a hard day and apply your own face mask. You know exactly what ingredients are in it and how sustainable or animal-friendly the products are. In a world that is constantly consuming and still pays far too little attention to resource-saving production, you can take the first step in the right direction for yourself and your bathroom by making your own cosmetic products simply and inexpensively.

For particularly sustainable products, you can use old and washed-out cream containers as packaging and simply reuse them again and again. For most cosmetic products, you do not need special packaging. You can also use leftover containers for mascara or lipsticks.

Vegan has also become a trend in cosmetics and, as is noted time and again, many of the recipes listed here are also vegan right from the start. However, if you want to have other recipes in vegan form, you can simply replace most of the ingredients with alternative products. For example, the milk can also be replaced by vegan almond or oat drinks, and there are now also numerous alternatives for honey or beeswax.

Making your own cosmetics is surprisingly easy and a lot of fun, especially with friends or family. It's insane when you compare how few ingredients a hand cream, a face mask or a hair shampoo make do with and how many additives can be found in the bought products. And these substances are often not only harmful to the environment, but your skin also suffers and can become additionally irritated or dried out. So, for your own sake, for the sake of the environment and animal welfare, decide to make your own cosmetic products and take half an hour now and then to make your own soap, make-up or shower gel.

Have fun!

Feel free to show off your homemade cosmetics, creams or deodorants!
Share a picture or video of your homemade product and post about it on Instagram.
Of course, don't forget to tag us so we can see & share your DIY item too!

You can find us on Instagram here:
https://www.instagram.com/mont.blonde/?hl=de

If you have any questions or similar, please don't hesitate to contact us on Instagram or at the following email address:

montblonde@outlook.com

Printed in Great Britain
by Amazon

37977336R00056